God's food heals

Piera Galvin

DISCLAIMER

THE INFORMATION IN THIS BOOK IS NOT TO BE USED
AS MEDICAL ADVICE AND IS NOT MEANT TO
TREAT OR DIAGNOSE MEDICAL PROBLEMS.
THE INFORMATION PRESENTED WITHIN SHOULD
BE USED IN COMBINATION WITH GUIDANCE
FROM YOUR DOCTOR.

THIS BOOK IS A PERSONAL JOURNEY
AND IS PRESENTED SOLELY FOR MOTIVATIONAL
AND INFORMATIONAL PURPOSES ONLY.

FIRST PUBLISHED – DECEMBER 2016

ISBN-10: 1541126270
ISBN-13: 978-1541126275

ALL SCRIPTURE QUOTATIONS ARE TAKEN FROM THE
AUTHORIZED VERSION KING JAMES HOLY BIBLE

VISIT MY WEBSITE AT:
WWW.GODSFOODHEALS.UK

CONTENTS

NEW YEAR'S EVE 2015

I was sitting up in bed writing to God in my journal, desperate for some help and guidance, because I really didn't think I was going to make it into 2016. You see, I had been struggling with my health for the past three years, and the doctor's just could not figure out what was wrong with me.

After spending a lot of money on private doctors and still not getting anywhere, I decided to go the alternative route, and saw a nutritionist and a homeopath. Both were really kind and understanding, and they advised me to have some tests done, so I did. The test results showed that my immune system was struggling, probably as a result of taking too many antibiotics in the past.

Internally, my body was a mess, and I now had a whole host of things wrong with me; Systemic Candida, Irritable Bowel Syndrome (IBS), Pelvic Adhesions, symptoms of Interstitial Cystitis (IC), and Coeliac Disease. I was losing weight fast, and that scared me more than anything. I will never forget the feeling of absolute despair I had that night when I cried out to God, pleading to Him to take this pain away from me, so that I could look after myself and my family.

The mistake I was making as a Christian was that I was trying to sort out my life by myself, and not bringing it to the Lord as He tells us to in His word, the Holy Bible. Therefore, after I had cried out to Him, I promised Him that I would study the foods in His word, as I believed with all my heart that He was the only One Who could guide me back to good health.

My husband has always said to me that *"ALL the answers to life are in the Bible"*, and it's absolutely true. God will always answer you if you are willing to study His word with an open heart.

During my journey, I have learned a lot about food and nutrition in general, using the Holy Bible as The Foundational Book. So within my humble little book here, you will read a combination of my personal testimony, Scripture verses I found, and some recipes I produced based on what I learned.

So I do hope and pray you enjoy reading this book, and take something from it that can help you in your life.

Piera Galvin
December 2016

THE ORIGINAL DIET

Genesis 1:11-12

And God said, Let the earth bring forth grass, the herb yielding seed, *and* the fruit tree yielding fruit after his kind, whose seed *is* in itself, upon the earth: and it was so. And the earth brought forth grass, *and* herb yielding seed after his kind, and the tree yielding fruit, whose seed *was* in itself, after his kind: and God saw that *it was* good.

Genesis 1:29-30

And God said, Behold, I have given you every herb bearing seed, which *is* upon the face of all the earth, and every tree, in the which *is* the fruit of a tree yielding seed; to you it shall be for meat. And to every beast of the earth, and to every fowl of the air, and to every thing that creepeth upon the earth, wherein *there is* life, *I have given* every green herb for meat: and it was so.

Genesis 2:9

And out of the ground made the LORD God to grow every tree that is pleasant to the sight, and good for food; the tree of life also in the midst of the garden, and the tree of knowledge of good and evil.

Abundant plant life

As we read in the scriptures, God has been looking after us right from the start, from the very beginning of creation.

He has provided us with an abundance of different foods, containing all the vitamins, minerals, and antioxidants our bodies need, in order to stay healthy.

But we have turned away from him, we have forgotten how to prepare and eat real wholesome food. With the excuses of having stressful, busy lives, we have turned to quick ready-made meals, which are high in fat, salt, and sugar, and devoid of any real nutrition.

After years of NOT eating properly and starving our bodies of the nutrients it so craves, our health starts to deteriorate and disease sets in. Then, the medication rollercoaster begins, with antibiotics, anti-inflammatories, steroid drugs, and so on.

I know that sometimes we just have to take them, for example a kidney infection that could be fatal if ignored, but there are so many natural alternatives out there, which can bring your body back into balance without the need for such man-made chemicals.

Pharmaceutical drugs can cause terrible side effects, which can lead to other health problems. Never getting to the root cause and only masking the problems. Therefore, the body never completely heals.

So, please listen to your body, because every disease is an indication that your body is missing something that it desperately needs.

It's never too late to improve your health. We just need to turn back to real food, and know that your body is a gift from God, and **is** capable of healing itself.

Eat More Veg!

Next time you sit down for a meal, take a good look at what is on your plate. Does it contain lots of brightly coloured vegetables and leafy greens, or maybe a big mixed salad? No, well it should, because all vegetables are anti-cancer and alkalizing, helping to keep our body's pH levels in balance, and free from disease.

So if your meals are lacking in colour, be creative. Perhaps stir fry some mixed peppers with onions, and enjoy with an egg or two. Make a nice rice and tuna salad with lots of freshly chopped cucumber, carrots, radish, sweet corn, red onion, and peppers, then squeeze some lemon juice and mix it through.

What's the easiest way to get your family eating all their vegetables? Yes, you guessed it! Put all the different vegetables into one pot, and make soups, stews, and casseroles for them. There you have it, problem solved!

'Cool as a Cucumber'

There were times when I just had to go to bed early. The relentless pain throughout my body would leave me physically and mentally drained. I would fall asleep instantly, only to be woken up in the middle of the night by what seemed to be a raging temperature due to the inflammation in my body.

Not wanting to disturb my husband by tossing and turning, and kicking off the bed covers, one morning I crept downstairs at 4 o'clock to make myself a herbal tea, and to read my Bible. Whilst reading, I came across Numbers chapter 11 verse 5, which reads, We remember the fish, which we did eat in Egypt freely; the cucumbers, and the melons, and the leeks, and the onions, and the garlick: Then suddenly, the thought 'cool as a cucumber' came to my mind.

I began to research the benefits of cucumber, and found that they are highly hydrating, and help detoxify the body, and lower inflammation. I was amazed! This was exactly what I needed to cool the heat from within my body. Now, I just had to wait for everyone else to wake up so that I could use my juicer to make a refreshing cucumber juice for breakfast.

And refreshing it was! We all enjoyed the juice, which contained 2 large organic cucumbers, and 1 large organic green apple (these are lower in sugar than the red ones).

Psalms 46:1
God is our refuge and strength,
a very present help in trouble.

RECIPE: Minestrone

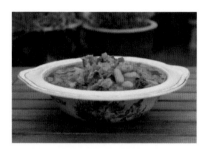

This minestrone is simple to make, and so good for you. I brought my children up on this dish, so that they would not and could not pick the vegetables out, because there were just too many of them. Now they love it!

Ingredients

Try and use organic produce whenever possible.

- 2 tablespoons of good quality olive oil
- 1 onion
- 2 garlic cloves – sliced
- 2 courgettes
- 2 carrots
- 2 celery sticks
- 1 large potato
- 1/2 savoy cabbage – core removed
- 100g green beans

- 2 gluten-free vegetable stock cubes (gluten-free and yeast-free if on a candida diet)
- 2 pints of hot boiled water
- 400g / 1 tin of chopped tomatoes
- 400g / 1 tin of cannellini or borlotti beans
- Season with 15 fresh basil leaves
- 1/2 teaspoon of dried oregano
- Salt and pepper

The above ingredients would serve 4 people.

How to make it

1. Prepare the vegetables – slice the onion and garlic, then set them aside.
2. Peel the carrots and the potato, then rinse them along with the courgettes, celery, cabbage, and green beans under cold running water.
3. Using a measuring jug, melt the stock cubes in 2 pints of hot boiled water.
4. In a medium-to-large saucepan, fry the sliced onion gently in the olive oil for a few minutes, until soft.
5. Then add the sliced garlic, and give it a stir.
6. Add in all the chopped vegetables, give it a good stir, and then add the tomatoes and the 2 pints of stock.

7. Season with the basil, oregano, and pepper (you may not need salt as the stock is already salty).

8. Bring to the boil then simmer for 1 hour 30 minutes to 2 hours, stirring from time to time.

9. Depending on how hard the beans are you may want to add them in about 30 minutes before the end of cooking.

If you would prefer to replace the cannellini or borlotti beans with pasta, you can snap 200g of gluten-free spaghetti into small pieces, cook separately, drain and add to the minestrone soup once it's cooked.

For me, minestrone is a comfort food; simple to make and super healthy.

THE CHANGED DIET

Animal Protein is Introduced

After the flood, the once perfect climate had now been disturbed.

Genesis 8:22
While the earth remaineth, seedtime and harvest, and cold and heat, and summer and winter, and day and night shall not cease.

This resulted in God instructing us to change our diet.

Genesis 9:3
Every moving thing that liveth shall be meat for you; even as the green herb have I given you all things.

It had now become essential for man to eat meat (animal protein), as well as the abundance of fruit and vegetables that God had given us, in order to protect and sustain our bodies from the ever changing weather.

We all need good quality protein to help build,

repair, and maintain muscular tissue in our body. But one thing I have to mention here is that when choosing your meat, make sure it is organic; the way God intended. Because unfortunately today, the majority of the animal protein that is sold to us has been injected with growth hormones and antibiotics. These then pass through the meat to us when we eat it, causing us many health problems.

Protein deficiency can affect any part of the body from hair loss to weight loss, infertility, anxiety, slow healing, and stiff joints. If you dislike eating meat, then there are many healthy and delicious high-protein alternatives to choose from, such as; cottage cheese, organic natural Greek yoghurt, eggs, quinoa, nuts and seeds, spinach, broccoli, and all types of beans.

I do eat mainly a vegetarian diet, but when I was having trouble with my digestive system, and everything that I was eating was going straight through me. My nutritionist advised me to eat a little more meat instead of all the high-fibre foods, as this would help me to regain my strength.

There are times when I really crave a piece of steak (organic, of course) with some peppercorn sauce (yum!), and I'm sure it's my body's way of saying, *"Hey, I need some protein to keep you going!"*

Oxen and Bovine Colostrum

1 Kings 19:21

And he returned back from him, and took a yoke of oxen, and slew them, and boiled their flesh with the instruments of the oxen, and gave unto the people, and they did eat. Then he arose, and went after Elijah, and ministered unto him.

Matthew 22:4

Again, he sent forth other servants, saying, Tell them which are bidden, Behold, I have prepared my dinner: my oxen and *my* fatlings *are* killed, and all things *are* ready: come unto the marriage.

Deuteronomy 14:4

These *are* the beasts which ye shall eat: the ox, the sheep, and the goat,

It was while studying oxen in the Bible, and doing some research on the benefits of eating organic beef, that I came across Bovine Colostrum.

This precious food is the pre-milk produced by cows for their calves. It is full of all the antibodies that they will need for life, and vital for their health, for without it they would become sick and die.

Four times stronger than human colostrum and

containing a myriad of health benefits, I was curious to know how it could help me. So after checking to see that the cows and their calves weren't harmed in any way while making it ready for human consumption, I decided to order some in powder form. I have also bought it in capsules for when I'm away from home.

The product I chose was Immune-Tree Colostrum 6. Known for *"Strengthening The Immune System. Supporting The Body's Renewal Process. Fortifying The Health of the GI Tract"*

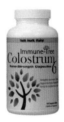

And it really does do what it says on the package!

Within 3 to 4 weeks of taking Bovine Colostrum, I noticed that my Irritable Bowel Syndrome (IBS) had calmed right down, enabling me to digest and absorb my food better. This was such a relief, because I had already lost 2-stone (28lbs) in weight over the past 3 months, and felt very weak all the time.

Then, within 9 months, the Interstitial Cystitis (IC – a debilitating bladder disease) symptoms that I also had, calmed down considerably, making it possible for me to *pee* every few hours instead of every hour.

The medical profession say that *"there is no cure"* for IC, but God is the **G**reat **P**hysician, and I would rather put my trust in Him!

Known as the first food of life, Bovine Colostrum has truly been an answer to prayer. I feel that God has given me a second chance at restoring my gut and everything else that was wrong with me.

If you're reading this and you have any type of gastrointestinal problems, whether it's Crohn's, IBS, Coeliac disease, etc., I hope and pray that you will also try this.

How I take Colostrum as a drink

- 1 to 2 tablespoons of Bovine Colostrum powder
- 1 glass of coconut or cashew milk (whichever your prefer)
- 1 level teaspoon of ground apricot kernels
- 1 or 2 inches of banana (NO banana if on a candida diet!)

Mix all the ingredients together in a blender until smooth, then drink as it is or pour over some sugar-free "crispy rice" or similar for a snack.

How I take Colostrum as capsules

Sometimes I will take 3 to 4 capsules twice a day with a glass of water, 20 minutes BEFORE a meal.

Please don't make the same mistake I made in the past! You take it, start feeling good, and then you stop. Just cut down your intake until you feel completely better.

<u>RECIPE: Italian-Style Burgers</u>

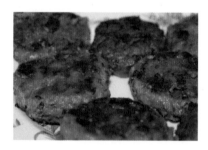

My parents have always used fresh breadcrumbs and Parmigiano-Reggiano cheese to make their delicious burgers. But because I am gluten intolerant, I skip the breadcrumbs and sometimes use Pecorino Romano cheese instead. This cheese is low in lactose, and may be suitable for those on a lactose-free diet.

My family and friends tell me the burgers taste just as nice, so I do hope you enjoy them too!

Ingredients

- 2 tablespoons of olive oil
- 4 tablespoons of gluten-free flour
  - For the meat mixture
    - About 400g to 500g of organic beef mince
- 2 eggs
- 3 heaped tablespoons of grated Parmesan cheese or Pecorino Romano cheese, if you're lactose intolerant
- 2 garlic cloves crushed or thinly sliced
- 20g or 2 tablespoons of fresh chopped parsley
- Salt and pepper for seasoning

The above ingredients would serve 3 to 4 people.

How to make it

1. Put the mince, eggs, Parmesan cheese, parsley, and garlic into a large bowl, and season with a little salt and pepper, and then mix all together with a fork until all combined.
2. Flour the surface of a large tray, and sprinkle a little flour over your hands, so that the meat mixture does not stick to them.

3. Scoop out a heaped tablespoon of meat mixture onto the floured surface, and mould into a burger shape.
4. Repeat until you get about 8 burgers, roughly 1cm thick and 7cm wide.
5. Put 2 tablespoons of oil into a large non-stick frying pan, and fry the burgers on a low-to-medium heat.
6. Press the burgers gently, and turn them over until golden and cooked through – should take about 15-20 minutes.

These are nice served with cooked green beans, drained, then tossed in a little extra virgin olive oil, sliced garlic, and sea salt. Tasty big salad and new potatoes.

<u>Sheep</u>

Deuteronomy 14:4

These *are* the beasts which ye shall eat: the ox, the sheep, and the goat,

1 Kings 4:22-23

And Solomon's provision for one day was thirty measures of fine flour, and threescore measures of meal, Ten fat oxen, and twenty oxen out of the pastures, and an hundred sheep, beside harts, and roebucks, and fallowdeer, and fatted fowl.

Nehemiah 5:18

Now *that* which was prepared *for me* daily *was* one ox *and* six choice sheep; also fowls were prepared for me, and once in ten days store of all sorts of wine: yet for all this required not I the bread of the governor, because the bondage was heavy upon this people.

Deuteronomy 32:14

Butter of kine, and milk of sheep, with fat of lambs, and rams of the breed of Bashan, and goats, with the fat of kidneys of wheat; and thou didst drink the pure blood of the grape.

<u>RECIPE: Stuffed Lamb Peppers</u>

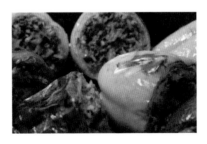

These peppers are really tasty, whether you eat them hot or cold. I usually serve mine with a big mixed salad, Feta cheese, and olives.

Ingredients

Makes 6 to 8 peppers, depending on their size.

- 126g wholegrain rice
- 2 tablespoons olive oil
- 240g lamb mince
- 6 to 8 peppers
- 1 cup of frozen Petit Pois peas
- 1/2 cup of Passata/ sieved or crushed tomatoes
- 3 heaped tablespoons of Parmesan cheese
- 1 heaped tablespoon of chopped fresh parsley or herb of your choice
- 1 large egg
- Salt and pepper for seasoning

The above ingredients would make 6 to 8 peppers, depending on size.

How to make them

1. In a saucepan, cook the rice, drain, and then set aside.
2. In a large frying pan, fry the sliced onion and garlic in the olive oil for a few minutes until soft.

3. Add the lamb mince, stir a little until sealed, and then add the peas.

4. Cut the tops off the peppers, discard the seeds and the stalks, BUT KEEP THE TOPS.

5. Set the peppers aside in an ovenproof dish.

6. Cut the tops of the peppers into small pieces, and add to the frying pan.

7. Add the Passata, parsley, and season with salt and pepper.

8. Cook all the ingredients together with a lid on for about 20 minutes, stirring from time to time. If the mixture is a little dry add a touch more Passata.

9. Take the frying pan off the heat and add the drained rice, mix together and bind with the egg and the Parmesan.

10. Using a tablespoon, scoop the mixture into the peppers and place back into the ovenproof dish. Drizzle a little olive oil over them, and place into the oven at Gas mark 6 or 200c, for about 30-45 minutes until they look soft and a little blistered.

Fish and Omega-3 Fatty Acids

Matthew 15:36

And he took the seven loaves and the fishes, and gave thanks, and brake *them*, and gave to his disciples, and the disciples to the multitude.

Luke 24:42

And they gave him a piece of a broiled fish, and of an honeycomb.

John 21:9-12

As soon then as they were come to land, they saw a fire of coals there, and fish laid thereon, and bread. Jesus saith unto them, Bring of the fish which ye have now caught. Simon Peter went up, and drew the net to land full of great fishes, an hundred and fifty and three: and for all there were so many, yet was not the net broken. Jesus saith unto them, Come *and* dine. And none of the disciples durst ask him, Who art thou? knowing that it was the Lord.

It is vital for our health and wellbeing to eat good quality foods containing Omega-3 fatty acids, as they consist of essential nutrients for our body.

These healthy fats can lower inflammation, reducing the risk of macular degeneration, Alzheimer's disease, arthritic pain, and depression.

They can also help with post menopausal symptoms by balancing the hormones.

You can find good sources of Omega-3 in wild-caught salmon, tuna, mackerel, herring, and sardines. But, saying that, I have to mention here that sadly we have to be cautious when buying fish, because some come from fish farms, and others from contaminated waters containing high levels of mercury. So next time you go shopping for fish, check to see where it comes from, or better still, visit your local harbour or fish market (if you live near any).

You can also get plant-based Omega-3 fatty acids in; dark green leafy vegetables, pecans, flaxseeds, hemp seeds, and chia seeds.

RECIPE: Cod in Tomato Sauce

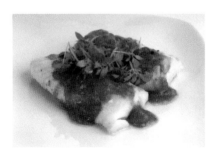

If I fancy something light for supper, I will normally cook a piece of fish, which I find easy to digest. I choose Cod as it works well with tomatoes, which adds colour to the dish (similar to the above photo).

This is lovely served with rice or new potatoes, along with some asparagus or broccoli. Or, steam some peas and sliced onions, and add a touch of olive oil.

Ingredients

- 4 pieces of cod (or other type of fish if your prefer)
- 2 tablespoons of olive oil
- 2 large vine tomatoes (ripe)
- 2 spring onions
- 1 garlic
- A little oregano, sea salt and pepper for seasoning

The above ingredients would serve 4 people.

How to make it

1. Slice the onions and garlic, and then fry gently in the olive oil until soft.
2. Chop the tomatoes into small pieces and add to the frying pan with a little oregano (about 1/2 teaspoon).

3. Fry for a few minutes until tomatoes just begin to soften.
4. Place the cod pieces into an ovenproof dish and pour the tomato sauce over them, season with salt and pepper.
5. Cover the dish with foil, and bake for about 20 minutes, (depending on the size of the fish), at 200c / Gas mark 6.

Lentils

Genesis 25:34

Then Jacob gave Esau bread and pottage of lentils; and he did eat and drink, and rose up, and went his way: thus Esau despised *his* birthright.

2 Samuel 17:28

Brought beds, and basons, and earthen vessels, and wheat, and barley, and flour, and parched *corn*, and beans, and lentils, and parched *pulse*,

Ezekiel 4:9

Take thou also unto thee wheat, and barley, and beans, and lentils, and millet, and fitches, and put them in one vessel, and make thee bread thereof, *according* to the number of the days that thou shalt lie upon thy side, three hundred and ninety days shalt thou eat thereof.

Daniel 1:12-16

Prove thy servants, I beseech thee, ten days; and let
them give us pulse to eat, and water to drink. Then
let our countenances be looked upon before thee,
and the countenance of the children that eat of the
portion of the king's meat: and as thou seest, deal
with thy servants. So he consented to them in this
matter, and proved them ten days. And at the end of
ten days their countenances appeared fairer and
fatter in flesh than all the children which did eat the
portion of the king's meat.

Lentils are wonderfully nutritious and considered to
be one of the world's healthiest foods. So next time
you make a soup or stew, don't forget to throw some
in.

RECIPE: Chicken and Lentil Stew

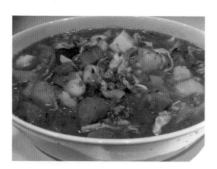

Ingredients

- 2 tablespoons of olive oil
- 4 large organic chicken thighs on the bone
- 1 large onion
- 3 large carrots
- 2 parsnips
- 3 medium to large potatoes (about 600g)
- 1/2 swede (about 235g)
- 2 gluten-free chicken stock cubes (if on a candida diet, use gluten-free, yeast free vegetable stock cubes instead)
- 2 pints of hot boiled water
- 1 tablespoon of chopped fresh parsley
- 400g / 1 tin of chopped tomatoes
- 400g / 1 tin of organic lentils
- Salt and pepper for seasoning (you may only need a little salt as the stock cubes are already salty)

The above ingredients would serve 5 to 6 people.

How to make it

You will need a large saucepan for this.

1. Slice onion thinly, then set aside.
2. Rinse, peel, and cut the carrots, parsnips, potatoes, and swede into 1-inch size pieces.
3. Remove the skin from the chicken thighs, and discard it.
4. Place the chicken thighs into the large saucepan with the olive oil, and fry gently for a few minutes until the meat is sealed.
5. Add the onion, stir a little, and then add all the chopped vegetables and the tin of tomatoes; continue cooking with the lid on.
6. Melt the stock cubes in the 2 pints of hot boiled water, and pour over the chicken and vegetables.
7. Add the parsley and season with some pepper.
8. Bring to the boil, and then cook on a low-to-medium heat, with the lid on for about 50 minutes.
9. Then add the lentils and cook for another 10-15 minutes.
10. After about 1 hour of cooking, check that the chicken is completely cooked through, by putting a fork through it. If the meat falls

off the bone then it's cooked, if not, allow to cook a little longer until the meat and vegetables are soft.

11. Once cooked, adjust seasoning, take chicken out, de-bone, and pop the meat back into the saucepan.

Serve with your favourite rice or hot gluten-free crusty rolls. Yum!

Beans

2 Samuel 17:28
Brought beds, and basons, and earthen vessels, and wheat, and barley, and flour, and parched *corn*, and beans, and lentiles, and parched *pulse*,

Ezekiel 4:9
Take thou also unto thee wheat, and barley, and beans, and lentiles, and millet, and fitches, and put them in one vessel, and make thee bread thereof, *according* to the number of the days that thou shalt lie upon thy side, three hundred and ninety days shalt thou eat thereof.

I really enjoy using beans in my recipes. They are reasonably inexpensive to buy, and come in all different colours, shapes, and sizes. They can 'bulk up' any meal, and make it super healthy and delicious.

My favourites are black beans, cannellini beans, barlotti beans, and lentils. We should all be eating more of these super healthy and delicious beans, especially if you don't eat meat. They are high in protein and rich in fibre, helping to keep you fuller for longer. They are also a good source of B-vitamins, which we all need in this stressful, busy world.

RECIPE: Black Bean Risotto

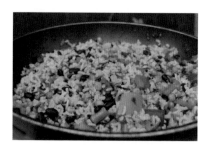

Ingredients

- 1 large tin of black beans
- 2 tablespoons of coconut oil
- 1 onion
- 1 large cup of garden peas
- 2 garlic cloves
- 1 tin of tomatoes (400g)

- 1 vegetable stock cube in 1 cup of boiled water (300ml)
- 125g of green beans
- 1 red pepper
- 1 green pepper
- Pepper (no salt)
- 1 tablespoon of fresh chopped parsley
- 1 cup of mixed brown basmati, red camargue and wild rice (cooked separately) – or use a rice of your choosing

The above ingredients would serve 4 people.

How to make it

1. Chop all the vegetables - onion, garlic, tomatoes, peppers, green beans, and parsley.
2. Put them into a bowl and set aside.
3. Melt the vegetable stock cube into a cup of hot boiled water, and set aside (you may want to start cooking the rice separately in a saucepan at this stage so that both dishes will be ready).
4. Pour 2 tablespoons of coconut oil into a large non-stick frying pan or wok.
5. Then add the onion and garlic, and fry gently for a few minutes.

6. Add all the chopped vegetables, including the cup of peas and vegetable stock, and season with pepper.
7. Cook on medium-to-low heat for about 30 to 45 minutes depending on how soft you like your vegetables.
8. Add black beans towards the end of cooking.
9. Then once everything is cooked, mix the rice through, and serve.

Rice

Being a very nutritious gluten-free grain, rice helps support the nervous system. It helps reduce the risk of heart disease by lowering cholesterol, and the fibre-rich content keeps the digestive system working properly.

The best rice to buy is black, brown, red, or wild. I tend to buy a bag of mixed rice and whole grain.

Oil of Olive

Deuteronomy 8:8
A land of wheat, and barley, and vines, and fig trees, and pomegranates; a land of oil olive, and honey;

Exodus 29:2
And unleavened bread, and cakes unleavened

tempered with oil, and wafers unleavened anointed with oil: *of* wheaten flour shalt thou make them.

Exodus 29:23

And one loaf of bread, and one cake of oiled bread, and one wafer out of the basket of the unleavened bread that *is* before the LORD:

My favourite oils have to be Extra Virgin Olive Oil, and coconut oil. These oils help decrease the risk of heart disease, cancer, and depression. They are also very good for balancing the hormones, and nourishing the skin and hair.

RECIPE: Olive Oil Salad Dressing

Ingredients

- 2 tablespoons of lemon juice or apple cider vinegar
- 2 tablespoons of extra virgin olive oil
- 1 teaspoon of dried oregano
- A little Himalayan salt or sea salt (a pinch)
- 1 crushed garlic clove

The above ingredients would serve 4 people.

How to make it

Mix all the ingredients together and pour over the salad.

I was the 'Queen' of salad dressings, sauces, and pickles; I couldn't eat a meal without one of them. Until I started the candida diet, and realised that these foods contain so much sugar.

Thank God I could still eat my olive oil salad dressing, which is so much healthier, and tastier too. So why not try and cut down on all those sauces you know you have tucked away in your fridge, and try this delicious version instead.

<u>Onions and Garlic</u>

Numbers 11:5

We remember the fish, which we did eat in Egypt freely; the cucumbers, and the melons, and the leeks, and the onions, and the garlick:

Onions and garlic have very powerful antifungal and antibacterial properties, which makes them great for keeping candida at bay, and fighting many other different types of infections.

Cheese & Dairy

1 Samuel 17:18

And carry these ten cheeses unto the captain of *their* thousand, and look how thy brethren fare, and take their pledge.

2 Samuel 17:29

And honey, and butter, and sheep, and cheese of kine, for David, and for the people that *were* with him, to eat: for they said, The people *is* hungry, and weary, and thirsty, in the wilderness.

Job 10:10

Hast thou not poured me out as milk, and curdled me like cheese?

Have you tried melting Feta cheese into pasta dishes, or sprinkling Pecorino Romano onto omelettes, and adding shavings of Parmigiano-Reggiano cheese to crispy salads? Yumm!

Not only do these cheeses taste great, but they are good for you too. They are easier to digest than many other cheeses, and promote the gut-friendly bacteria 'Bacillus Bifidus' that we could all have more of in these days.

RECIPE: Simple Feta Salad

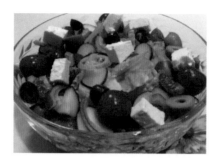

I love using Dolce Verde Romaine Hearts in my salads, because they are so crisp and sweet. All the vegetables in this salad have many health benefits. They are full of enzymes, which aid in digestion, and they are also very good at reducing inflammation in the body, and are full of antioxidants.

This salad makes a great side dish. I could eat this salad every night, but not without my olive oil salad dressing.

Ingredients

- About 100g of Feta cheese
- 2 small Dolce Verde Romaine Hearts
- 130g cherry tomatoes
- 1 small red pepper
- 1/2 red onion
- 1 small cucumber
- 5 radishes

- 2 to 3 tablespoons of olives

The above ingredients would allow 4 people to share.

How to make it

1. Rinse and slice the Romaine Hearts (I use a salad spinner to get rid of the excess water, but a good shake in the colander is fine), and place into a large salad bowl.
2. Cut and slice all the other vegetables, and add to the bowl with the olives.
3. Make up olive oil salad dressing (for recipe, see page 37).
4. Pour it over and mix it through.
5. Crumble the Feta cheese over the salad or cut into slices, and then serve.

These are the cheeses I use most:

- Feta (made from sheep or goats milk, or a combination of both)
- Pecorino Romano (made from sheep and goats milk)
- Parmigiano-Reggiano (made from cows milk)

These cheeses are a good source of calcium, which supports bone health. They are easier to digest than many other cheeses, and promote the gut-friendly bacteria, 'Bacillus Bifidus', and you will only need a little in your recipes, as they are big on flavour.

Eggs

Job 6:6
Can that which is unsavoury be eaten without salt?
or is there *any* taste in the white of an egg?

Luke 11:12
Or if he shall ask an egg,
will he offer him a scorpion?

Praise the Lord, I am not allergic to eggs; my family and I absolutely love them.

Eggs kept me going, while on a candida diet, and I would have them poached, boiled, scrambled or fried almost every morning. I would serve them with, sliced avocados, grilled or fresh tomatoes and spinach.

Sometimes I would really fancy some organic bacon and gluten-free sausages too. I replaced the gluten-free bread, (because it contains yeast) with sweet potato flatbread, and they taste so good.

I got the sweet potato flatbread (roti) recipe from a video on YouTube.

I CAN EAT SWEET THINGS AGAIN!

Numbers 13:23

And they came unto the brook of Eshcol, and cut down from thence a branch with one cluster of grapes, and they bare it between two upon a staff; and *they brought* of the pomegranates, and of the figs.

2 Kings 20:7

And Isaiah said, Take a lump of figs. And they took and laid *it* on the boil, and he recovered.

Song of Solomon 2:5

Stay me with flagons, comfort me with apples: for I *am* sick of love.

Song of Solomon 7:8

I said, I will go up to the palm tree, I will take hold of the boughs thereof: now also thy breasts shall be as clusters of the vine, and the smell of thy nose like apples;

Song of Solomon 7:12

Let us get up early to the vineyards; let us see if the vine flourish, *whether* the tender grape appear, *and* the pomegranates bud forth: there will I give thee my loves.

Song of Solomon 2:13

The fig tree putteth forth her green figs, and the vines *with* the tender grape give a *good* smell. Arise, my love, my fair one, and come away.

Oh how I would love to have seen Solomon's garden in the springtime. It must have been so picturesque with all the fruit trees in blossom.

Childhood memories come to mind of our summer holidays in Italy. My sisters and I loved to run up and down my Nonna's orchard, picking lusciously sweet figs straight off the trees.

Why not replace some of those chocolates, cakes, and biscuits that all offer little or no nutritional value whatsoever, with fresh fruit that is bursting with vitamins and minerals. Their powerful antioxidants can reduce the risk of cancer, high blood pressure, constipation, and acne.

So put that 'body destroying food' away, and grab an apple instead!

Nuts

Genesis 43:11

And their father Israel said unto them, If *it must be* so now, do this; take of the best fruits in the land in your vessels, and carry down the man a present, a little balm, and a little honey, spices, and myrrh, nuts, and almonds:

Numbers 17:8

And it came to pass, that on the morrow Moses went into the tabernacle of witness; and, behold, the rod of Aaron for the house of Levi was budded, and brought forth buds, and bloomed blossoms, and yielded almonds.

Song of Solomon 6:11

I went down into the garden of nuts to see the fruits of the valley, *and* to see whether the vine flourished, *and* the pomegranates budded.

Whenever I mention nuts, my friends often say, *"Oh, but they're fattening"*. Well, they're not as fattening as that piece of cake you're having every night with your cup of tea! No, nuts are very nutritious, and they all offer different health benefits.

When I'm feeling peckish, I'll often have a pot of natural Greek yogurt with some chopped green apple, and some lightly roasted mixed nuts with a drizzle of honey. Now that's so much nicer and healthier than a piece of cake!

Raisins

1 Samuel 25:18
Then Abigail made haste, and took two hundred loaves, and two bottles of wine, and five sheep ready dressed, and five measures of parched *corn*, and an hundred clusters of raisins, and two hundred cakes of figs, and laid *them* on asses.

1 Samuel 30:12
And they gave him a piece of a cake of figs, and two clusters of raisins: and when he had eaten, his spirit came again to him: for he had eaten no bread, nor drunk *any* water, three days and three nights.

2 Samuel 16:1
And when David was a little past the top *of the hill*, behold, Ziba the servant of Mephibosheth met him, with a couple of asses saddled, and upon them two hundred *loaves* of bread, and an hundred bunches of raisins, and an hundred of summer fruits, and a bottle of wine.

1 Chronicles 12:40

Moreover they that were nigh them, *even* unto
Issachar and Zebulun and Naphtali, brought bread
on asses, and on camels, and on mules, and on oxen,
and meat, meal, cakes of figs, and bunches of raisins,
and wine, and oil, and oxen, and sheep abundantly:
for *there was* joy in Israel.

Genesis 40:10-11

And in the vine *were* three branches: and it *was* as
though it budded, *and* her blossoms shot forth; and
the clusters thereof brought forth ripe grapes: And
Pharaoh's cup *was* in my hand: and I took the grapes,
and pressed them into Pharaoh's cup, and I gave the
cup into Pharaoh's hand.

After studying these verses, I came to the conclusion
that there really is no need to keep using white
processed or any other colour sugar, when baking
cakes.

Many years ago they sweetened their cakes using
dried fruit, nuts, and honey, so I attempted to make
a sugar free banana cake and it came out surprisingly
sweet.

RECIPE: Sugar-Free Banana Cake

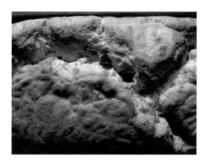

I don't really have a sweet tooth and I've never really been a big fan of desserts, but I have to admit that whenever my husband and I go out to a restaurant, I just have to have a little bit of his dessert and this drives him crazy – I'm sure it's a man thing you know, not wanting to share desserts!

Anyway, this banana fruitcake is a real treat; moist, tasty, and sweet enough without sugar. What could go wrong? Well a lot really. It almost drove me crazy trying to get it to rise.

So after many failed attempts, and almost putting myself off bananas altogether, I've discovered that gluten-free flour can be very tricky and doesn't rise like other flours.

I find it's best to keep your ingredients, such as eggs, butter and flour at room temperature, and check that your baking powder is still fresh.

This is a nice treat for when the children get home from school, instead of watching them raid the cupboards looking for chocolate, crisps and biscuits, as they often like to do.

Ingredients

- 245g gluten-free self raising flour
- 1 teaspoon of baking powder
- 2 large eggs at room temperature
- 85g unsalted butter – melted
- 200ml coconut milk (or milk of your choice)
- 2 ripe bananas – mashed
- 50g sultanas
- 50g chopped dried pitted dates
- 1 tablespoon of runny honey

The above ingredients would serve up to 6 people. This is based on cutting slightly larger slices, as gluten-free cakes tend to crumble easier than a gluten cake.

How to make it

1. Grease and line a loaf tin, 900g (216) in size.
2. Sift flour and baking powder together into a mixing bowl.

3. In a separate bowl, mix the melted butter, eggs and milk together.
4. Add the wet ingredients to the flour, and stir gently until well combined.
5. Then fold the mashed bananas, sultanas, dates and honey gently into the cake mixture.
6. Pour the cake mixture into the loaf tin and bake at 180c / 350f / Gas mark 4, for 1 hour.

Try not to open the oven door for a peek while it's baking, because it will sink. After an hour, check the cake by putting a knife through it. The knife should come out clean. Leave to cool completely before slicing, and enjoy with your favourite herbal tea. Also, absolutely lovely with custard!

<u>Honey</u>

Proverbs 16:24

Pleasant words *are as* an honeycomb, sweet to the soul, and health to the bones.

Proverbs 24:13

My son, eat thou honey, because *it is* good; and the honeycomb, *which is* sweet to thy taste:

Numbers 14:8

If the LORD delight in us, then he will bring us into

this land, and give it us; a land which floweth with milk and honey.

Luke 24:42
And they gave him a piece of a broiled fish,
and of an honeycomb.

Rowse Cut Comb In Acacia Honey is delightfully sweet, and 100% pure and natural. It boosts the immune system, and wards off infection.

I like to spread it on toast, drizzle over pancakes, stir it into porridge, and add it to fruit and yoghurt.

RECIPE: Fruit and Yoghurt

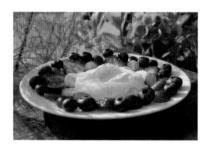

Ingredients

I used two handfuls.

- Blueberries
- Red grapes
- Strawberries

- 2 bananas
- 4 small pots of organic natural Greek yoghurt
- 1 teaspoon of honey with a slither of honeycomb

The above ingredients would serve 4 people.

How to make it

1. Rinse and drain the blueberries, grapes, and strawberries.
2. Slice the bananas, and cut the grapes and strawberries in half.
3. Arrange the fruit nicely around the plate, and pour the yoghurt in the centre.
4. Drizzle a teaspoon of honey over the fruit, and finish off with a slither of honeycomb on the yoghurt.

Organic Natural Greek Yoghurt

If you look after your gut, your gut will look after you! So make time to enjoy natural Greek yoghurt, which is packed with probiotics to help keep you strong and healthy.

CANDIDA

Well, how can I explain it? Let me put it like this. Candida Albicans as it's known, affects people in different ways, making it difficult to identify the problems they are suffering from.

But for me, it was like a silent invasion; a slow burning fire, sweeping through my body, causing inflammation, and attacking my weakest organs, which happened to be my kidneys and my bladder.

I couldn't even manage working a few hours as a hairdresser in a care home. Instead of me looking after the elderly, they would be comforting me! I couldn't wait to get home for my husband to rub my back. My pelvis, and the whole of my body felt like it was in a vice.

Then, the panic attacks started, which I had never experienced before in my life. They would come and go for what seemed like absolutely no reason whatsoever. It was a very frightening experience, and all due to an overgrowth of yeast; a fungus, which normally lives in the body with no problem.

You see, problems arise when the body's

immune system has been compromised in some way. Whether it's through eating a high carbohydrate diet of white bread, pasta, and rice, or chocolates, cakes, and biscuits. Not to mention the sugar-laden fizzy drinks, which really stress the body. These foods have been stripped of any real nutrition, and are 'fuel' for candida.

Or maybe, like me, you have taken too many antibiotics or other pharmaceutical drugs in the past, and have never replaced your gut with good quality probiotics. This has then left you open and vulnerable to all sorts of intestinal problems, such as Leaky Gut Syndrome, IBS, Crohn's, Coeliac disease, and many more.

It is essential for you to replace the beneficial bacteria in your gut. You can do this by eating unsweetened organic natural yoghurt, and taking a good quality probiotic, which is kept in the fridge. You could also add Kefir, and fermented foods to your diet, once your candida levels are back to normal (a homeopath can test you for this).

Even constantly worrying and being negative about life can affect you terribly. When you don't feel well, it's difficult to 'snap out of it', but you have to try, for you and your family's sake.

The Scripture that I find really helpful is in Mathew chapter 11 verses 28 to 30, where Jesus says:

Come unto me, all *ye* that labour and are heavy laden, and I will give you rest. Take my yoke upon you, and learn of me; for I am meek and lowly in heart: and ye shall find rest unto your souls. For my yoke *is* easy, and my burden is light.

There is NO greater comfort than the word of God! None! He knows exactly how you feel, and what you need. If you haven't read the Bible in a while, then I encourage you to start right away.

You could also try and spend some quality time with friends and family. Or if you prefer, you could do something for yourself, such as joining an exercise class, writing, painting, cooking, sewing – there's so much out there; we just have to be willing to change and stay positive.

Not realising that you have gluten intolerance, and eating the wrong foods can put your immune system under great strain.

Grains containing gluten are wheat, rye, barley, spelt, and sometimes oats (unless stated as gluten-free oats). These grains have been genetically modified (GM), and I don't believe that they are suitable for human consumption anymore. They are not what God originally gave us, and are now toxic to our bodies, causing many health complications.

Once you start replacing those grains with healthier alternatives, such as; buckwheat, quinoa, rice, amaranth, millet, corn, sorghum, and teff, you will find that your immune system will strengthen, and you will have a lot more energy.

WATER AND SALT

Genesis 26:19

And Isaac's servants digged in the valley, and found there a well of springing water.

Exodus 17:6

Behold, I will stand before thee there upon the rock in Horeb; and thou shalt smite the rock, and there shall come water out of it, that the people may drink. And Moses did so in the sight of the elders of Israel.

Numbers 20:8

Take the rod, and gather thou the assembly together, thou, and Aaron thy brother, and speak ye unto the rock before their eyes; and it shall give forth his water, and thou shalt bring forth to them water out of the rock: so thou shalt give the congregation and their beasts drink.

Deuteronomy 8:7

For the LORD thy God bringeth thee into a good land, a land of brooks of water, of fountains and depths that spring out of valleys and hills;

Deuteronomy 11:11

But the land, whither ye go to possess it, *is* a land of hills and valleys, *and* drinketh water of the rain of heaven:

Judges 1:15

And she said unto him, Give me a blessing: for thou hast given me a south land; give me also springs of water. And Caleb gave her the upper springs and the nether springs.

<u>Water</u>

I have to say, I am terrible when it comes to drinking water. I just don't drink enough of it; I'd rather have a herbal tea instead. Well herbal teas are supposed to be good for you, aren't they?

But after looking deeply at these Scriptures, I have come to realise just how important and necessary pure water is. Our entire body, EVERY cell depends on it. No amount of herbal tea or any other beverage is ever going to replace the essential minerals that are found in pure natural spring water. So, from now on I'm going to remind myself to drink pure water, by carrying a bottle of spring water with me wherever I go.

Word of caution – avoid bottled water that includes fluoride.

One of my favourite verses in God's word is John chapter 4 verse 10, which reads: Jesus answered and said unto her, If thou knewest the gift of God, and who it is that saith to thee, Give me to drink; thou wouldest have asked of him, and he would have given thee living water.

Salt

Ezra 6:9
And that which they have need of, both young bullocks, and rams, and lambs, for the burnt offerings of the God of heaven, wheat, salt, wine, and oil, according to the appointment of the priests which *are* at Jerusalem, let it be given them day by day without fail:

Job 6:6
Can that which is unsavoury be eaten without salt? or is there *any* taste in the white of an egg?

Luke 14:34
Salt *is* good: but if the salt have lost his savour, wherewith shall it be seasoned?

Matthew 5:13

Ye are the salt of the earth: but if the salt have lost his savour, wherewith shall it be salted? it is thenceforth good for nothing, but to be cast out, and to be trodden under foot of men.

Believe it or not, but salt is good and is essential to life! However, NOT the regular table salt you normally find in cafés, restaurants, and at your local supermarket. No, that unhealthy 'version' is highly processed, devoid of minerals, and contains anti-caking agents and chemicals. This is far from the salt that God blessed us with.

Real salt, such as Himalayan Pink Crystal Rock Salt, contains 84 minerals, which help to support all our bodily functions. And it tastes great too! Here are just some benefits from eating this salt:

- Supports proper digestion, the nervous system, adrenal glands, and the metabolism
- Promotes stable pH balance in the cells.

- Alleviates muscle cramps.
- Normalises blood sugar.

God has provided us with the best salt on earth! Once you've tried it, you will never want to go back to any man-made, chemical-laden salt again.

You should be able to find this real salt in your health food store, or you can order it online. I am actually going to start carrying in my purse a small vial of this salt for whenever I eat out.

GETTING BACK INTO BALANCE

I shudder at the thought of how much pain and discomfort I was in a year ago. Having a combination of Interstitial Cystitis, Irritable Bowel Syndrome, Pelvic adhesions, Systemic candida, and Coeliac disease, made my 'insides' feel raw and inflamed.

As you can imagine, car journeys became difficult and almost unbearable at times, forever needing to go to the toilet as the pressure from my IC would make me feel as though I had a constant bladder infection. My only comforts were; D-mannose, which I would take every 2-3 hours until the bladder spasms calmed down, and a doughnut-ring seat cushion to sit on.

Holidays and weekends away were cut short. Meals out with friends and family were cancelled, and all because anxiety and panic attacks would keep me from leaving the comfort of my own house.

But these 'fiery trials' have kept me close to the Lord, and with His help, guidance, and strength, I was massively determined to find natural alternatives to better health.

He is lifting me out of this physical 'mire' that I

have been in, and as I write this, I feel so much happier and healthier than I have been in a long time.

I hope and pray that you (or someone you talk to) will be blessed by reading this little book.

The Steps I Took

As I mentioned earlier, I found a very good nutritionist who advised me to have a comprehensive stool test done. This enabled us to see what was going on in my gut and intestines. The test results showed severe intestinal candida (overgrowth of yeast), and that I didn't have any of the beneficial bacteria, called Lactobacillus, in my gut.

Therefore I had to try and starve the candida by going on a strict diet for a while of no dairy, yeast, wheat or sugar, and that also included fruit.

I took the antifungal, Caprylic Acid, Olive Leaf Extract and Grapefruit Seed Extract, which I found only helped me while I was on them.

I drank lots of different herbal teas and vegetable juices, and ate lots of immune-boosting foods, such as onions and garlic (I felt sorry for my husband!) every night.

I cooked with turmeric, ginger, and coconut oil, even eating it straight off the spoon.

I also took 14 vitamins a day to support my immune system, and a probiotic high in Lactobacillus to repopulate my gut with the good bacteria.

But after four months of doing this diet, I was still loosing weight, in pain and feeling very weak and tired. So my nutritionist, who was very professional, thought that I might be suffering with Leaky Gut Syndrome, caused by the candida, and kindly recommended that I see someone about a food sensitivity test.

Desperately searching and praying for some help, God revealed Bovine Colostrum to me, while studying the foods in the Bible. Within three to four weeks of taking this food supplement my Irritable Bowel Syndrome had finally calmed down, and I began putting weight on, and my energy levels picked up.

Then 4 months later I found a wonderful homeopath. She used the Vega Test machine, and tested me for allergies and food sensitivities, and candida.

The Vega Test revealed that I was allergic to

wheat, rye, barley, spelt, malt, vinegar, bitter, and lager. Well, the last two didn't bother me as I didn't drink any alcohol, but the others did.

Being Italian, I thought, *"How am I going to live without my bread and pasta!?"*, and as for the candida, that was still severe. At least now I knew what was wrong with me, and I could finally do something about it.

So this time, my candida problem only took 16 weeks to clear up as I had Colostrum on my side, strengthening and repairing my gut.

I took the advice of my homeopath and armed myself with lots of information on Coeliac disease. I cleared all my kitchen cupboards of any gluten ingredients, just incase I accidently used any while cooking, and then stocked up on all the healthy gluten-free grains, flours, nuts, and seeds.

My husband decided to surprise me one day by booking me in with a personal trainer for 10 exercise sessions. I couldn't believe it; I had never been one for 'jumping around up and down', and my idea of exercise was walking round the shops and cleaning the house. But I have to say that after each session I felt much better, and with every passing week I grew in stamina. Now I use a re-bounder when I feel up to it, and my Pilates DVD to keep me lengthened, strengthened, and toned.

As I'm coming towards the end of this book, I have only one more health problem to sort out, praise God, and that's my pelvic adhesions.

This scar-like tissue developed after having two Caesarean sections (C-sections), and a couple of cysts that had burst on my ovaries.

I believe that these bands of scar tissue have wrapped themselves around my ovaries, bladder, and bowel, and are causing the interstitial cystitis symptoms I experience. I say symptoms, because I refused to have a doctor insert a camera inside my bladder to check it and stretch it at the same time, only for them to then send me home with yet more antibiotics, and the possibility of bladder incontinence.

I have spent almost a year trying different therapies in the hope of sorting this problem out, without having to go 'under the knife'. I've had Deep Tissue Massage, and Swedish Massage. I've been to see a Chiropractor, and also tried Bowen Technique Therapy, which I did find really relaxing and calming to my nerves. But even though they were all good, they could only help me up to a point.

I really needed someone who would actually focus on loosening the scar tissue around my C-section.

One morning, my husband and I decided to go food shopping together. I was walking down an aisle when suddenly the pain around my pelvis grew so intense that uncontrollable tears streamed down my face. Embarrassed and helpless, I rushed back to the car, and my husband drove us home.

Feeling low and running out of ideas as to what to do next, unbeknownst to me, my husband was already searching online for yet another therapist. It didn't take him long at all. He walked into the room where I was sitting, and said, *"I've booked an appointment for you. I think she's the one. She's a massage therapist who works on C-section adhesions."* I was so grateful, and couldn't wait for my appointment.

As I write this, it has been 5 weeks since my husband made that appointment, and I've had 3 deep tissue massage sessions so far. The first was terribly painful, but desperately needed as the therapist worked hard at loosening the scar tissue around my pelvis. She could feel a hard lump just under my C-section, and thought that this was probably the cause of most of my bladder and bowel problems.

Once the session was over, I felt cold, tender, and bruised. My husband said that my body was perhaps in shock after having been 'disturbed' so much during the massage. Whatever the case, I wondered whether I had made a mistake by getting it done. However, a few days later, once the swelling had gone down, I felt as though my pelvic organs had been 'released', and I could move freely.

The second session did not hurt as much, and the third one was surprisingly comfortable. The lump and surrounding scar tissue she had worked on had finally softened, and it has made such a difference to my life.

During this time, we received a gift of some essential oils from our wonderful friends over in America. This got me thinking about how I could apply essential oils to my body by massaging my scar tissue area. After a bit of research, I settled on 'Frankincense' for its healing properties (and also because it was given to the young child Jesus so it must be great!).

I started to massage 4 drops of Frankincense oil mixed with 1 large teaspoon of melted organic coconut oil onto my pelvic area and tummy every night for 1 week. I was astonished at how fast this stuff works! The Frankincense oil is truly special, and has amazing healing properties, which help protect the immune system from inflammation, pain, and disease.

Knowing this, and also inhaling its pleasant aroma, I find it really helps me to unwind and sleep so much better, giving my body the necessary and needed time to repair and strengthen itself.

As I type this, it is December 2016 and I can happily say that I am feeling so much better than I have in the last 3 years. Although I will probably always be on a gluten-free diet (which isn't actually a bad thing!), the IC has gone, the IBS has gone, and the candida has gone. Praise the Lord!

EXAMPLE SHOPPING LIST

Here's a quick review of some of the foods that I have used and mention in this little book. They are listed/grouped in alphabetic order, and include a brief look at their nutritional benefits.

Apple Cider Vinegar

☐ Bragg Organic

Is a good way of getting more probiotics into your gut. The acetic acid it contains destroys harmful bacteria, and promotes the beneficial ones; keeping your digestive tract healthy.

Animal protein

☐ Beef
☐ Chicken
☐ Eggs
☐ Lamb

We need to eat good quality, organic meat, to help build, repair, and maintain muscular tissue in our body.

Calcium

- ☐ Feta (made from sheep or goats milk, or a combination of both)
- ☐ Pecorino Romano (made from sheep and goats milk)
- ☐ Parmigiano-Reggiano (made from cows milk)

Supports bone health. These cheeses are easier to digest than many others, and promote the gut-friendly bacteria 'Bacillus Bifidus'. You will only need a little in your recipes, as they are big on flavour.

Cod

The Omega-3 fatty acids found in fish, can help protect the heart and brain, and also reduce inflammation throughout the body.

Dairy-Free Milk

- ☐ Koko Dairy Free

"Made from freshly pressed coconut milk."

"Naturally free of lactose, cow's milk protein, soya or gluten intolerance."

"Nut free and packed in a nut free environment, Coconuts are a fruit not a nut."

"Suitable for Vegans, Vegetarians, and Coeliacs"

"Cholesterol free and with Calcium and fat levels matched to semi-skimmed milk."

"Fresh tasting and versatile to use in drinks and in cooking."

"GMO Free."

Always check ingredients when buying other coconut dairy-free alternatives, as they may contain nuts.

☐ Alpro Cashew Milk Original

"Low in Sugars"

"Naturally Low in Fat"

"Easy to digest as naturally lactose free"

"Free from dairy and gluten"

"Free from Colours and flavours"

"Suitable for Vegans"

"May Contain: Nuts"

Fruit

☐ Bananas
☐ Blueberries
☐ Dried Pitted Dates
☐ Red Grapes
☐ Strawberries
☐ Sultanas

Contain powerful antioxidants that can help reduce

the risk of cancer, high blood pressure, constipation, and acne.

Herbs

- ☐ Basil
- ☐ Oregano
- ☐ Parsley

Powerful antibacterial properties, and packed full of vitamins and minerals.

Honey

- ☐ Rowse Cut Comb in Acacia Honey

Delightfully sweet and 100% pure and natural. Boosts the immune system and wards off infection.

Oils

- ☐ Coconut Oil
- ☐ Extra Virgin Olive Oil
- ☐ Olive Oil and Olives

Help decrease the risk of heart disease, cancer, and depression. Also very good for balancing the hormones, and nourishing the skin and hair.

Organic Natural Greek Yoghurt

Packed with probiotics to help keep you strong and healthy.

Organic Tinned Beans

- ☐ Black Beans
- ☐ Borlotti Beans
- ☐ Cannellini Beans
- ☐ Lentils

High in protein, and rich in fibre. Good source of B Vitamins.

Rice

- ☐ Black
- ☐ Brown
- ☐ Red
- ☐ Wild
- ☐ or buy a bag of mixed rice and whole grain

Helps support the nervous system, reduces the risk of heart disease by lowering cholesterol, and the fibre-rich content keeps the digestive system working properly.

Vegetables

- ☐ Cabbage
- ☐ Carrots
- ☐ Celery
- ☐ Courgettes
- ☐ Cucumber
- ☐ Green Beans
- ☐ Lemon
- ☐ Lettuce – Dolce Verde Romaine Hearts
- ☐ Parsnips
- ☐ Peppers (Bell)
- ☐ Petit Pois Garden Peas
- ☐ Potatoes
- ☐ Radishes
- ☐ Swede/rutabaga
- ☐ Tomatoes

Anti-cancerous and alkalizing, helping to keep your body's pH levels in check.

Vegetables - Allium

- ☐ Brown Onion
- ☐ Garlic
- ☐ Red Onion
- ☐ Spring Onion

Onions, guaranteed to make you cry, but they're

worth it as they have very powerful antifungal and antibacterial properties, which help fight many different types of infections. So try and get these wonderful aromatic foods into your diet as much as possible.

Other ingredients I used:

- ☐ Gluten-free self raising flour
- ☐ Gluten-free chicken stock cubes
- ☐ Gluten-free, and yeast-free vegetable stock cubes
- ☐ Sea salt or Himalayan salt
- ☐ Black pepper
- ☐ Organic unsalted butter
- ☐ Organic tin of tomatoes

HAVE THESE IN YOUR CUPBOARD

As well as the products I have already mentioned, I would also recommend having the following items readily available to you:

Bitter Apricot Kernels

Bitter apricot kernels are rich in vitamin B17, and very nutritious.

Plagued with ovarian cysts on and off over the years, I decided to do some research, and found many testimonies of people healing themselves from cancers, tumours, and cysts using B17. So I took the recommended amount of apricot kernels for my weight in pounds, and within one month my cyst had shrunk, relieving some of the pressure and pain on my left ovary and bladder.

Vitamin B17 is also found in; cashew nuts, macadamia nuts, apple seeds, and kernels of peaches, cherries, and plums.

Colloidal Silver

Colloidal Silver is great for eliminating infections. I used to dread the winter months, as I would almost always come down with tonsillitis. But last year, I was ready and waiting with this little silver spray bottle by my side.

One night, I awoke with a terrible sore throat, and found it very difficult to swallow. So I quickly sprayed my throat with the colloidal silver wanting to stop the soreness developing into full-blown tonsillitis. In the morning I felt much better, so I continued with the spraying every few hours for a couple of days, and it cleared up completely without any need for over-the-counter medicine or antibiotics.

Bicarbonate of Soda

This helps to reduce the acidity in the urine, but don't do this to often as it can raise blood pressure.

Sweet Cures Waterfall D-mannose

When I had candida, and I ate foods containing gluten (without realising I was a Coeliac), my bladder would react by going into terrible spasms.

Whether it was a Urinary Tract Infection (UTI) or not, I wasn't going to wait for it to get any worse. So I would take the recommended amount of D-mannose (which is 100% natural), to flush away any 'nasty, unwanted' bacteria from my bladder, without the need for antibiotics. This stuff is amazing!

PEOPLE WHO HAVE INSPIRED ME

Here are the names of some men and women who the Lord led me to over the years, and who have really helped me through their videos, books, articles, and lectures:

- Dr John Bergman
- Dr Josh Axe
- Charlotte Gerson
- Dr Tulio Simoncini
- Dr Leonard Coldwell

I would highly recommend visiting their websites and/or YouTube channels. You will be greatly blessed!

GOD AND HIS SALVATION

I have always tried to see the 'good' in people, and I still do. But while studying God's word, the Holy Bible, the Lord has taught me so much, and truly opened my eyes and understanding to what we have done to this precious planet.

We have brought sickness and disease upon ourselves through selfishness and greed. We have depleted our soil, genetically modified our food, contaminated our waters, and polluted the air we breathe. It's no wonder then why you or someone you know is suffering from some type of illness.

But God is merciful; always watching over us and guiding us. And He continually provides for us the essential foods and drink that can help us to lead and maintain the best physical life we can on this earth.

<u>Are you saved?</u>

We must remember though that this physical life we all have will end one day no matter how healthy we become. And the question then for all of us is, *"Where will we spend eternity?"*

The Holy Bible says that there is only ONE WAY to Heaven, and that is by the Lord Jesus Christ (God in the flesh), who said, I am the way, the truth, and the life: no man cometh unto the Father, but by me.

God says that we have all sinned against Him, and that we need to have our sins forgiven before He can allow us into Heaven. No amount of 'good works' we do can ever get us there. God says that we need to believe the gospel that the Lord Jesus Christ died for our sins, was buried, and rose again on the third day. If we BELIEVE this with our hearts, trusting Him ALONE for salvation, then God says that we will be SAVED, and Heaven is our home when we die.

Won't you call on Him TODAY to receive His forgiveness! Pray from your heart, and ask God to forgive you of your sins, and accept the sacrifice that the Lord Jesus Christ made for you.

A BIG THANK YOU

Below is a list of people I would like to personally thank, who have really helped me over these last couple of years.

- God (without Him I wouldn't even be alive! He is first in <u>everything</u>)
- My husband and two beautiful daughters
- Church family (for their support and prayers)
- Mum and Dad (for their love of food!)
- Our neighbour, Bill (for providing me with organic produce)
- Jacob and Mary Elizabeth (for their prayers and essential oils)
- And the professional therapists; Auriol, Mandy, Christine, Lee, Sadie, and Jane.

Thank you so much for reading my little book!

Please visit my website at:

www.GodsFoodHeals.uk

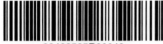

29482585R00048

Printed in Great Britain
by Amazon